THE
INSULIN SOLUTION

How to manage your blood sugar and take back your health

Esther C. Excel

Table of contents

INTRODUCTION

Welcome to "The Insulin Solution: Taking Control of Your Blood Sugar". This book is your comprehensive guide to understanding insulin, blood sugar, and the powerful connection between the two. It's a journey that will empower you to take charge of your health, transform your life, and unlock the secrets of insulin wisdom.

Imagine waking up every morning feeling refreshed, revitalized, and ready to tackle the day. Your energy levels are soaring, your mind is clear, and your body is thriving. You're in control of your health, and your blood sugar levels are perfectly balanced.

But for many of us, this is just a distant dream. We struggle with mysterious weight gain, fatigue, mood swings, and a never-ending cycle of blood sugar highs and lows. We feel like we're losing control of our bodies, and the medical professionals seem to be speaking a language we can't understand.

That's exactly what happened to Sarah, a vibrant 35-year-old marketing executive who thought she had it all together. She was active, ate well, and loved trying new restaurants and practicing yoga. But beneath the surface, Sarah was struggling. She felt tired all the time, her weight was creeping up, and her mood swings were becoming more frequent.

One fateful day, Sarah's doctor delivered a life-changing diagnosis: type 2 diabetes. The news shook her to her core. She had always associated diabetes with her grandparents' generation, not her own. As she grappled with the reality of her new condition, Sarah felt overwhelmed by the sheer amount of information and advice thrown her way.

Determined to take charge of her health, Sarah embarked on a journey to understand insulin and its role in her body. She devoured books, attended seminars, and consulted with experts. But the more she learned, the more she realized how complex and nuanced insulin management could be.

Sarah's story is not unique. Millions of people worldwide struggle to manage their insulin levels, often feeling frustrated, defeated, or simply unsure of where to start. But what if there was a way to break free from the cycle of confusion and take control of your insulin health?

That's where "The Insulin Solution" comes in – a comprehensive guide to understanding insulin, blood sugar, and the powerful connection between the two. Through a combination of scientific research, real-life examples, and practical strategies, this book will empower you to:

- Understand the fascinating world of insulin and its impact on your body

- Develop a personalized plan to manage your insulin levels and improve your overall health

- Navigate the often-confusing landscape of nutrition, exercise, and medication

- Build resilience and confidence in the face of challenges and setbacks

Over the next pages, we'll delve into the intricate dance between insulin and blood sugar, exploring the latest scientific discoveries and translating them into actionable advice. We'll meet inspiring individuals who have transformed their lives by mastering insulin management, and we'll break down complex concepts into accessible, bite-sized pieces.

"The Insulin Solution" is more than just a book – it's a roadmap to reclaiming your health, your energy, and your life. Join me on this journey, and discover the transformative power of insulin wisdom. Let's take the first step towards unlocking the secrets of insulin and taking control of your blood sugar, once and for all.

CHAPTER ONE: UNDERSTANDING INSULIN AND BLOOD SUGAR

The Insulin Story: How it Works and Why it Matters

As we embark on this journey to understand insulin and blood sugar, let's start with the fascinating story of insulin itself. Like a master key, insulin unlocks the doors to our cells, allowing glucose to enter and provide energy for our bodies. But how does it work, and why is it so crucial for our health?

Imagine a bustling city, where glucose is the fuel that powers the vehicles. Insulin is the traffic cop, directing the flow of glucose into the cells, ensuring that the city runs smoothly and efficiently. Without insulin, the city would come to a grinding halt, and the vehicles would stall.

In the early 20th century, Canadian researchers Frederick Banting and Charles Best discovered insulin, revolutionizing the treatment of diabetes. They found that insulin is produced in the pancreas, a small organ located behind the stomach, and is released into the bloodstream to regulate blood sugar levels.

Here's how it works:

- After a meal, carbohydrates are broken down into glucose, which enters the bloodstream.

- The pancreas detects the rise in blood glucose levels and releases insulin.
- Insulin binds to receptors on the surface of cells, unlocking the doors and allowing glucose to enter.
- Cells use glucose for energy, growth, and repair.
- As glucose enters the cells, blood sugar levels decrease, and the pancreas reduces insulin production.

But why is insulin so important? Without it, glucose builds up in the bloodstream, causing a range of problems, from mild discomfort to life-threatening complications. Insulin's role extends beyond just regulating blood sugar levels; it also:

- Helps regulate fat storage and metabolism
- Influences hormone production and balance
- Affects cognitive function and mood

The insulin story is one of the vital hormones that plays a central role in our overall health. By understanding how insulin works and why it matters, we can begin to appreciate the complex relationships between insulin, blood sugar, and our bodies.

Blood Sugar Basics: Understanding the Numbers and the Impact

As we continue our journey to understand insulin and blood sugar, it's essential to grasp the basics of blood sugar itself. What is blood sugar, and why is it so crucial for our health? In this chapter, we'll delve into the world of blood sugar, exploring the numbers, the impact, and the delicate balance that keeps our bodies thriving.

Meet Emma, a 28-year-old graphic designer who loves baking and trying new recipes. Emma was recently diagnosed with prediabetes, and her doctor told her to monitor her blood sugar levels regularly. But what did those numbers mean, and how would they impact her life?

Blood sugar, also known as blood glucose, is the amount of glucose present in our bloodstream. Glucose is a type of sugar that serves as our body's primary source of energy. When we eat, carbohydrates are broken down into glucose, which enters the bloodstream, triggering the release of insulin.

Here's a key concept: blood sugar levels are measured in milligrams per deciliter (mg/dL). A normal fasting blood sugar level is typically below 100 mg/dL. After a meal, blood sugar levels may rise, but they should return to normal within a few hours.

The insulin solution

Now, let's explore the different blood sugar ranges and their impact on our health:

- Normal blood sugar: Below 100 mg/dL
- Prediabetes: 100-125 mg/dL
- Diabetes: 126 mg/dL or higher

But what happens when blood sugar levels become imbalanced? Let's examine the effects of high and low blood sugar:

High Blood Sugar (Hyperglycemia):

- Fatigue and weakness
- Increased thirst and urination
- Blurred vision
- Slow healing of cuts and wounds

Low Blood Sugar (Hypoglycemia):

- Shakiness and dizziness
- Sweating and confusion
- Hunger and irritability
- Seizures (in severe cases)

Emma learned that managing her blood sugar levels was crucial to preventing long-term complications, such as nerve damage, kidney disease, and vision problems. She began to monitor her levels regularly, using a glucometer to track her progress.

Remember, blood sugar basics are just the beginning. As we continue this journey, you'll gain a deeper understanding of the intricate relationships between insulin, blood sugar, and your body.

CHAPTER TWO: THE SCIENCE OF INSULIN MANAGEMENT

Insulin Types and Timing: Finding the Right Balance

As we delve into the science of insulin management, it's essential to understand the different types of insulin and their timing. Imagine a symphony orchestra, where each musician plays a unique instrument, working together in harmony to create a beautiful melody. Similarly, various insulin types work together to regulate blood sugar levels, and timing is crucial to achieve perfect harmony.

Meet David, a 42-year-old entrepreneur who has lived with type 1 diabetes for over two decades. David has tried various insulin regimens, but he still struggles to find the right balance. He experiences highs and lows, affecting his energy levels and overall well-being.

There are several types of insulin, each with a distinct duration of action:

1. Rapid-acting insulin (aspart, lispro, glulisine): Starts working within 15 minutes, peaks in 1-2 hours, and lasts for 2-4 hours.

2. Short-acting insulin (human insulin): Starts working within 30 minutes, peaks in 2-3 hours, and lasts for 4-6 hours.

3. Intermediate-acting insulin (NPH): Starts working within 2-4 hours, peaks in 4-12 hours, and lasts for 12-18 hours.
4. Long-acting insulin (glargine, detemir): Starts working within 2-4 hours, has a flat peak, and lasts for 20-24 hours.

5. Ultra-long-acting insulin (degludec): Starts working within 1-4 hours, has a flat peak, and lasts for 42 hours.

David's healthcare provider explained that finding the right balance of insulin types and timing is crucial to managing his blood sugar levels effectively. They worked together to develop a personalized plan, taking into account David's lifestyle, diet, and activity level.

Here's a key concept: insulin stacking. When taking multiple injections, it's essential to space them out to avoid overlapping peaks, which can cause hypoglycemia. For example, if David takes rapid-acting insulin before breakfast, he should wait at least 2-3 hours before taking intermediate-acting insulin.

In addition to insulin types and timing, other factors influence blood sugar control, such as:

- Carbohydrate counting: Understanding how different foods affect blood sugar levels.

- Insulin-to-carbohydrate ratio: Determining the optimal insulin dose based on carbohydrate intake.

- Correction factor: Adjusting insulin doses to correct high blood sugar levels.

By mastering insulin types, timing, and these additional factors, David achieved better blood sugar control, reducing his highs and lows. He felt more energetic, focused, and in control of his diabetes.

Nutrition and Insulin: How Food Affects Blood Sugar

As we continue our journey through the science of insulin management, it's time to explore the fascinating world of nutrition and its impact on blood sugar levels. Imagine a master chef, expertly combining ingredients to create a culinary masterpiece. Similarly, our bodies are constantly balancing the ingredients we consume, using insulin to regulate blood sugar levels.

Maria is a 35-year-old fitness enthusiast who has struggled with weight management and blood sugar swings. She loves trying new recipes but often finds herself feeling lethargic and bloated after meals. Maria's healthcare provider suggested she examine her nutrition choices and their impact on her insulin sensitivity.

Carbohydrates, protein, and fat – the three main macronutrients – affect blood sugar levels in unique ways. Let's break down each:

- Carbohydrates: Broken down into glucose, causing blood sugar levels to rise. Simple carbs (sugar, white bread) cause a rapid spike, while complex carbs (whole grains, vegetables) lead to a more gradual increase.

- Protein: Stimulates insulin release, but also helps regulate blood sugar levels. Protein-rich foods like lean meats, fish, and eggs can improve insulin sensitivity.
- Fat: Slows down carbohydrate digestion, reducing the impact on blood sugar levels. Healthy fats like avocado, nuts, and olive oil support insulin function.

Maria learned that understanding glycemic index (GI) and glycemic load (GL) was crucial to managing her blood sugar levels. GI measures how quickly a food raises blood sugar, while GL takes into account the serving size.

- Low GI/GL foods: Whole grains, non-starchy vegetables, and most fruits

- Medium GI/GL foods: Whole grain bread, brown rice, and sweet potatoes

- High GI/GL foods: White bread, sugary snacks, and refined grains

By incorporating low GI/GL foods and balancing her macronutrient intake, Maria noticed significant improvements in her energy levels and blood sugar control. She felt empowered to make informed choices, knowing that her nutrition decisions directly impacted her insulin sensitivity.

In addition to macronutrients and GI/GL, other nutritional factors influence blood sugar levels:

- Fiber: Delays carbohydrate digestion, reducing blood sugar spikes

- Water intake: Essential for insulin function and blood sugar regulation

- Omega-3 fatty acids: Supports insulin sensitivity and reduces inflammation

By mastering the intricate relationships between nutrition, insulin, and blood sugar, Maria achieved a deeper understanding of her body's needs. She continued to explore new recipes, but now with a newfound appreciation for the impact of food on her overall health.

Exercise and Insulin Sensitivity: Moving Towards Better Health

As we continue our journey through the science of insulin management, it's time to explore the dynamic relationship between exercise and insulin sensitivity. Imagine a powerful engine, with exercise serving as the spark that ignites the fuel of insulin, driving our bodies toward better health.

Jack is a 50-year-old entrepreneur who has struggled with type 2 diabetes for over a decade. Despite his best efforts, Jack's blood sugar levels remained stubbornly high, and he felt like he was losing control. His healthcare provider suggested he incorporate exercise into his daily routine, but Jack was skeptical. He had tried before but found it difficult to stick to a program.

However, Jack's provider explained that exercise is a potent tool for improving insulin sensitivity, allowing glucose to enter cells more efficiently. Regular physical activity can:

- Increase glucose uptake in muscles
- Enhance insulin signaling pathways
- Reduce inflammation and oxidative stress

Intrigued, Jack began with short walks during his lunch break and gradually progressed to more intense workouts. He discovered that exercise not only improved his blood sugar control but also boosted his energy levels and overall well-being.

Let's delve deeper into the science behind exercise and insulin sensitivity:

- Aerobic exercise: Activities like brisk walking, cycling, and swimming improve cardiovascular health and increase insulin sensitivity.

- Resistance training: Building muscle mass through weightlifting or bodyweight exercises enhances glucose uptake and insulin signaling.

- High-intensity interval training (HIIT): Short bursts of intense exercise followed by brief rest periods have been shown to improve insulin sensitivity and cardiovascular health.

As Jack continued his exercise journey, he noticed significant improvements in his blood sugar control. His healthcare provider explained that regular physical activity had:

- Increased his muscle mass, allowing for more efficient glucose uptake

- Enhanced his insulin signaling pathways, improving insulin sensitivity
- Reduced his inflammation and oxidative stress, lowering his risk of chronic diseases

The insulin solution

In addition to exercise, other lifestyle factors influence insulin sensitivity:

- Stress management: Chronic stress can reduce insulin sensitivity; engage in stress-reducing activities like yoga or meditation

- Sleep quality: Poor sleep can disrupt insulin function; aim for 7-8 hours of sleep per night

- Social connections: Building strong relationships can improve mental health and insulin sensitivity

By incorporating exercise and other lifestyle modifications, Jack achieved remarkable improvements in his blood sugar control and overall health. He felt empowered, knowing that his daily choices directly impacted his insulin sensitivity and well-being.

CHAPTER THREE: PRACTICAL SOLUTIONS FOR INSULIN MANAGEMENT

Creating a Personalized Insulin Plan: Setting Goals and Tracking Progress

As we embark on this journey to master insulin management, it's essential to create a personalized plan that suits your unique needs and goals. Imagine a roadmap, guiding you through the twists and turns of insulin management, helping you navigate the challenges and celebrate the triumphs.

Sarah is a 30-year-old marketing specialist who has struggled with type 1 diabetes since childhood. Despite her best efforts, Sarah's blood sugar levels remained unpredictable, and she felt like she was constantly playing catch-up. She knew she needed a personalized plan to take control of her insulin management.

Sarah's healthcare provider helped her set specific, achievable goals:

The insulin solution

- Improve blood sugar control, reducing highs and lows

- Increase physical activity, aiming for 30 minutes of exercise
per day

- Develop a balanced meal plan, focusing on whole foods and
portion control

Together, they created a personalized insulin plan, taking into
account Sarah's:

- Lifestyle and schedule
- Dietary preferences and restrictions
- Physical activity level and goals
- Insulin sensitivity and needs

Sarah learned to track her progress, using a combination of:

- Blood glucose monitoring
- Food and exercise logs
- Insulin dose tracking

By monitoring her progress, Sarah identified patterns and
trends, making adjustments to her plan as needed. She
celebrated small victories, like mastering a new exercise
routine or trying a new recipe.

Let's break down the key components of a personalized
insulin plan:

The insulin solution

- Goal setting: Identify specific, achievable objectives, such as improving blood sugar control or increasing physical activity

- Insulin dosing: Determine the optimal insulin doses and timing, based on individual needs and lifestyle

- Meal planning: Develop a balanced meal plan, taking into account dietary preferences and restrictions

- Physical activity: Incorporate regular exercise, aiming for at least 150 minutes of moderate-intensity activity per week
- Tracking and monitoring: Regularly track progress, using tools like blood glucose monitoring, food and exercise logs, and insulin dose tracking

In addition to these components, other factors influence insulin management:

- Stress management: Chronic stress can impact blood sugar control; engage in stress-reducing activities like yoga or meditation

- Sleep quality: Poor sleep can disrupt insulin function; aim for 7-8 hours of sleep per night

- Social support: Build a support network of family, friends, and healthcare providers to help navigate challenges

By creating a personalized insulin plan and tracking progress, Sarah achieved remarkable improvements in her blood sugar control and overall health. She felt empowered, knowing that her daily choices directly impacted her insulin management and well-being.

Mastering Insulin Dosing: Tips and Strategies for Success

As we continue our journey to master insulin management, it's essential to develop a deep understanding of insulin dosing. Imagine a skilled artist, carefully balancing colors and textures to create a masterpiece. Similarly, mastering insulin dosing requires a delicate balance of timing, dosage, and adjustments to achieve optimal blood sugar control.

Emily is a 25-year-old artist who has lived with type 1 diabetes since childhood. Despite her best efforts, Emily struggled with insulin dosing, often experiencing highs and lows. She felt like she was constantly guessing, trying to find the perfect balance.

Emily's healthcare provider taught her the fundamentals of insulin dosing:

- Understanding insulin types: rapid-acting, short-acting, intermediate-acting, and long-acting

- Calculating insulin doses: based on carbohydrate intake, physical activity, and blood sugar levels

The insulin solution

- Timing insulin doses: coordinating with meals, exercise, and sleep

Emily learned to fine-tune her insulin dosing, using the following tips and strategies:

- Start with a basal dose: a small, steady dose of insulin throughout the day

- Add bolus doses: before meals and snacks, based on carbohydrate intake

- Adjust for physical activity: increasing or decreasing doses based on exercise intensity and duration

- Consider correction doses: for high blood sugar levels, using a correction factor

By mastering insulin dosing, Emily achieved remarkable improvements in her blood sugar control. She felt confident, knowing that she had the skills to adjust her doses and navigate challenges.

Let's delve deeper into the world of insulin dosing, exploring advanced strategies for success:

- Insulin-to-carbohydrate ratio: determining the optimal insulin dose based on carbohydrate intake

- Insulin sensitivity factor: adjusting doses based on individual insulin sensitivity

- Dual-wave dosing: using a combination of rapid-acting and short-acting insulin for optimal coverage

In addition to these strategies, other factors influence insulin dosing:

- Hormonal changes: adjusting doses during menstruation, pregnancy, or menopause

- Travel and time zones: considering time changes and adjusting doses accordingly

- Illness and stress: increasing doses during times of illness or stress

By mastering insulin dosing and considering these factors, Emily achieved optimal blood sugar control and improved her overall health. She felt empowered, knowing that she had the skills to manage her insulin and live a vibrant life.

Overcoming Common Challenges: Troubleshooting and Adjusting

As we navigate the complex world of insulin management, challenges will inevitably arise. Imagine a skilled navigator, charting a course through treacherous waters. Similarly, overcoming common challenges in insulin management requires skill, patience, and persistence.

Rachel is a 40-year-old business owner who has lived with type 2 diabetes for over a decade. Despite her best efforts, Rachel encountered a series of challenges that left her feeling frustrated and defeated.

- Unpredictable blood sugar swings
- Insulin resistance and decreased sensitivity
- Difficulty losing weight and maintaining weight loss
- Frequent hypoglycemic episodes

Rachel's healthcare provider helped her identify the root causes of these challenges and develop strategies to overcome them.

- Unpredictable blood sugar swings: Adjusting insulin doses and timing, and incorporating physical activity to improve insulin sensitivity.

- Insulin resistance and decreased sensitivity: Focusing on weight loss, increasing physical activity, and optimizing nutrition.

- Difficulty losing weight and maintaining weight loss: Developing a personalized meal plan, incorporating strength training, and addressing emotional eating habits.
- Frequent hypoglycemic episodes: Adjusting insulin doses and timing, and carrying emergency glucose supplies.

By troubleshooting and adjusting her approach, Rachel overcame these challenges and achieved optimal blood sugar control. She felt empowered, knowing that she had the skills to navigate any obstacle.

Let's explore additional common challenges and strategies for overcoming them:

- Dealing with insulin pump issues: Troubleshooting technical problems, and developing a backup plan for insulin delivery.

- Managing diabetes during travel: Researching destination-specific diabetes resources, and packing essential supplies.

- Coping with emotional challenges: Building a support network, practicing stress-reducing techniques, and seeking professional help when needed.

In addition to these strategies, other factors can impact insulin management:

- Hormonal fluctuations: Adjusting insulin doses and timing during menstruation, pregnancy, or menopause.

- Medication interactions: Coordinating with healthcare providers to minimize potential interactions.

- Lifestyle changes: Adjusting insulin doses and timing during periods of significant change, such as retirement or moving.

By understanding common challenges and developing effective troubleshooting strategies, Rachel achieved a deeper understanding of her insulin management needs. She felt confident, knowing that she could overcome any obstacle and maintain optimal blood sugar control.

CHAPTER FOUR : TAKING CONTROL OF YOUR HEALTH

Mindset and Motivation: Staying on Track with Your Insulin Plan

As we journey through the world of insulin management, it's essential to acknowledge the profound impact of mindset and motivation on our ability to stay on track. Imagine a skilled athlete, fueled by determination and focus, pushing through challenges to achieve victory. Similarly, cultivating a strong mindset and motivation is crucial to overcoming obstacles and achieving success in insulin management.

Meet Michael, a 35-year-old entrepreneur who has lived with type 1 diabetes since childhood. Despite his best efforts, Michael struggled to maintain a consistent insulin plan, often finding himself derailed by stress, anxiety, and frustration.

Michael's healthcare provider encouraged him to explore the power of mindset and motivation, recognizing that a positive and resilient mindset is essential to achieving optimal insulin management.

- Setting realistic goals: Breaking down large goals into smaller, achievable milestones

- Building self-awareness: Recognizing thought patterns, emotions, and behaviors that impact insulin management
- Cultivating self-compassion: Practicing kindness, understanding, and patience when faced with challenges

- Developing a growth mindset: Embracing challenges as opportunities for growth and learning

By adopting this mindset and motivation framework, Michael transformed his approach to insulin management. He:

- Developed a consistent insulin plan, tailored to his unique needs and lifestyle

- Improved his blood sugar control, reducing highs and lows

- Enhanced his overall well-being, experiencing increased energy and confidence

Let's delve deeper into the world of mindset and motivation, exploring additional strategies for success:

- Visualization techniques: Imagining success and achievement to boost motivation

- Positive self-talk: Encouraging oneself with affirmations and supportive language

- Accountability partnerships: Sharing goals and progress with a trusted friend or mentor

- Reward systems: Celebrating milestones and achievements with non-food rewards

In addition to these strategies, other factors can impact mindset and motivation:

- Social support: Surrounding oneself with encouraging and understanding individuals

- Self-care: Prioritizing activities that bring joy and relaxation

- Mindfulness: Practicing present-moment awareness to reduce stress and increase focus

By cultivating a strong mindset and motivation, Michael achieved a profound shift in his approach to insulin management. He felt empowered, knowing that he had the tools to overcome any obstacle and maintain optimal blood sugar control.

We'll explore the importance of ongoing learning and growth in insulin management, examining how staying up-to-date with the latest research and technologies can help you achieve optimal wellness. By embracing a commitment to lifelong learning, you'll be empowered to navigate the ever-evolving landscape of insulin management with confidence and success.

Building a Support Network: Surrounding Yourself with Help and Encouragement

As we journey through the world of insulin management, it's essential to recognize the profound impact of a support network on our ability to thrive. Imagine a skilled team, working together in harmony to achieve victory. Similarly, surrounding yourself with a supportive community is crucial to overcoming challenges and achieving success in insulin management.

Sophia is a 28-year-old artist who has lived with type 2 diabetes for several years. Despite her best efforts, Sophia struggled to maintain a consistent insulin plan, often feeling isolated and alone in her journey.

Sophia's healthcare provider encouraged her to build a support network, recognizing that a strong community is essential to achieving optimal insulin management.

- Family and friends: Educating loved ones about diabetes and insulin management, and asking for their support

- Support groups: Joining online or in-person communities to connect with others who share similar experiences

The insulin solution

- Healthcare providers: Building a strong relationship with healthcare professionals, and seeking their guidance and support

- Online resources: Utilizing reputable online forums, blogs, and educational platforms to stay informed and connected

By building a support network, Sophia transformed her approach to insulin management. She:

- Felt less isolated, knowing that she had a community of understanding and encouragement

- Gained valuable insights and advice from others who shared similar experiences

- Developed a more positive mindset, recognizing that she was not alone in her journey

- Improved her blood sugar control, reducing highs and lows

Let's delve deeper into the world of support networks, exploring additional strategies for success:

- Identifying support network roles: Recognizing the unique contributions of each network member

- Building a support network plan: Developing a plan for regular check-ins and communication

- Navigating challenging relationships: Setting boundaries and prioritizing self-care when faced with unsupportive individuals

- Celebrating milestones: Acknowledging and celebrating achievements with support network members

In addition to these strategies, other factors can impact support networks:

- Cultural and linguistic diversity: Recognizing the importance of culturally sensitive support networks

- Accessibility and inclusivity: Ensuring that support networks are accessible and inclusive for all individuals

- Technology and social media: Leveraging technology to connect with support networks and access resources

By building a strong support network, Sophia achieved a profound shift in her approach to insulin management. She felt empowered, knowing that she had a community of help and encouragement surrounding her.

We will explore the importance of ongoing learning and growth in insulin management, examining how staying up-to-date with the latest research and technologies can help you achieve optimal wellness. By embracing a commitment to lifelong learning, you'll be empowered to navigate the ever-evolving landscape of insulin management with confidence and success.

Thriving with Insulin: Long-Term Success and Wellness

As we conclude our journey through the world of insulin management, it's essential to focus on the ultimate goal: thriving with insulin and achieving long-term success and wellness. Imagine a vibrant garden, flourishing with lush greenery and colorful blooms. Similarly, thriving with insulin requires nurturing and attention, but the rewards are immeasurable.

Daniel is a 45-year-old entrepreneur who has lived with type 1 diabetes for over two decades. Despite the challenges, Daniel has thrived with insulin, achieving optimal blood sugar control and living a vibrant life.

Daniel's journey to thriving with insulin was not without its obstacles. He faced:

- Burnout and frustration: Feeling overwhelmed by the demands of insulin management

- Fear and anxiety: Worrying about long-term complications and the impact on his life

- Self-doubt and shame: Struggling with feelings of inadequacy and guilt

However, Daniel persevered, and with the help of his healthcare provider, he developed strategies for long-term success:

- Setting realistic goals: Breaking down large goals into smaller, achievable milestones

- Building resilience: Developing coping skills and learning to adapt to challenges
- Cultivating self-awareness: Understanding his thoughts, emotions, and behaviors and their impact on insulin management

- Nurturing self-care: Prioritizing activities that bring joy and relaxation

By implementing these strategies, Daniel achieved:

- Optimal blood sugar control: Reducing highs and lows and minimizing complications

- Improved overall health: Enhancing his physical and mental well-being

- Increased confidence: Feeling empowered and in control of his insulin management

- Enhanced quality of life: Living a vibrant and fulfilling life, free from the constraints of diabetes

The insulin solution

Let's explore additional strategies for thriving with insulin:

- Staying up-to-date: Embracing new technologies and research to optimize insulin management

- Building a legacy: Sharing knowledge and experience with others to inspire and educate

- Embracing community: Connecting with others who share similar experiences to build support and connection
- Celebrating milestones: Acknowledging and celebrating achievements along the journey

In addition to these strategies, other factors can impact long-term success:

- Healthcare provider relationships: Building strong, collaborative relationships with healthcare professionals

- Family and friend support: Surrounding oneself with encouraging and understanding loved ones

- Personal growth: Embracing challenges as opportunities for growth and self-improvement

By thriving with insulin, Daniel achieved a profound shift in his approach to diabetes management. He felt empowered, knowing that he had the tools and strategies to live a vibrant and fulfilling life.

Remember that thriving with insulin is a lifelong path. By embracing the strategies and mindset outlined in this book, you'll be empowered to navigate the ever-evolving landscape of insulin management with confidence and success.

CONCLUSION

Putting it All Together: Your Path to Insulin Success

As we conclude our journey through the world of insulin management, it's essential to reflect on the transformative power of knowledge, mindset, and community. Imagine a majestic tapestry, woven from threads of understanding, resilience, and connection. Similarly, your path to insulin success is a unique and intricate journey, requiring patience, dedication, and support.

Throughout this book, we've explored the complexities of insulin management, from the science of insulin to the art of thriving with insulin. We've met individuals who have faced challenges and overcome obstacles, emerging stronger and more resilient.

As you embark on your path to insulin success, remember that:

- Knowledge is power: Understanding insulin, nutrition, and physical activity is crucial to making informed decisions

- Mindset matters: Cultivating a positive, resilient mindset is essential to navigating challenges and setbacks

- Community is key: Surrounding yourself with support, encouragement, and connection is vital to long-term success

By embracing these principles, you'll be empowered to:

- Take control of your insulin management

- Develop a personalized plan that suits your unique needs and goals

- Build a strong support network of healthcare providers, loved ones, and peers

- Thrive with insulin, achieving optimal blood sugar control and overall wellness

As you move forward, remember that your path to insulin success is unique, and it's okay to encounter twists and turns. Don't be afraid to ask for help, seek guidance, and learn from others.

In the words of our journey's companions:

- "Insulin management is a journey, not a destination. Be patient, stay curious, and keep moving forward." - Rachel

- "Community is the unsung hero of insulin success. Surround yourself with people who uplift and support you." - Daniel

- "Knowledge is the foundation of empowerment. Keep learning, growing, and adapting to achieve optimal insulin management." - Sophia

As you close this book, remember that your path to insulin success is just beginning. Embrace the journey, stay committed, and know that you are not alone.

In the final words of our journey, we leave you with a sense of hope, empowerment, and connection. May your path to insulin success be illuminated with knowledge, guided by resilience, and supported by the community.

Congratulations, you've taken the first step towards thriving with insulin. Now, go forth and live a vibrant, fulfilling life, unencumbered by the constraints of diabetes.

APPENDIX

Additional Resources - Tools, Templates, and References for Further Learning

As we conclude our journey through the world of insulin management, we recognize that learning is a lifelong process. To support your continued growth and exploration, we've curated a comprehensive appendix of additional resources, tools, and templates.

Tools and Templates

1. Insulin Management Tracker: A customizable template to monitor blood sugar levels, insulin doses, and physical activity.

2. Meal Planning Worksheet: A practical tool to plan balanced meals and snacks, taking into account carbohydrate counting and portion control.

3. Exercise Log: A template to track physical activity, including duration, intensity, and type.

4. Stress Management Journal: A reflective tool to identify and manage stressors, emotions, and coping strategies.

5. Medication Adherence Chart: A simple template to track medication schedules and doses.

References for Further Learning

1. American Diabetes Association (ADA) - A comprehensive resource for diabetes management, including research, education, and advocacy.

2. Centers for Disease Control and Prevention (CDC) - A trusted source for diabetes information, including statistics, guidelines, and resources.

3. Joslin Diabetes Center - A renowned organization offering diabetes education, research, and clinical care.

4. Mayo Clinic - A respected healthcare provider offering expert advice and resources on diabetes management.

5. National Institute of Diabetes and Digestive and Kidney Diseases (NIDDK) - A government-funded organization providing research, education, and resources on diabetes and related conditions.

Online Communities and Forums

1. Diabetes Forum - A supportive online community for people living with diabetes, offering discussion forums, blogs, and resources.

2. Insulin Nation - An online platform providing news, education, and community for people affected by diabetes.

3. TuDiabetes - A social network for people living with diabetes, offering forums, blogs, and resources.

Mobile Apps

1. mySugr - A comprehensive diabetes management app, that tracks blood sugar levels, medication, and physical activity.

2. OneDrop - A user-friendly app for tracking blood glucose, medication, and food intake.

3. Glucose Buddy - A simple app for tracking blood sugar levels, medication, and physical activity.

Books and Publications

1. "The Diabetes Bible" by Dr. Joseph P. Napora - A comprehensive guide to diabetes management, covering nutrition, exercise, and medication.

2. "Insulin Pump Therapy" by Dr. John Walsh - A practical guide to insulin pump management, covering basics, advanced features, and troubleshooting.

3. "Diabetes Burnout" by Dr. William H. Polonsky - A thought-provoking book exploring the emotional and psychological aspects of diabetes management.

By leveraging these additional resources, you'll be empowered to continue learning, growing, and thriving with insulin. Remember, knowledge is power, and community is key. Stay connected, stay informed, and stay committed to your path to insulin success.